DR. SANDRA JIMASON

CERTIFIED LIFE COACH
& SPIN INSTRUCTOR

FAT TO FIT AT FIFTY+

TACKLING EMOTIONAL AND MENTAL
BARRIERS TO WEIGHT LOSS

A HEALTHY WEIGHT LOSS GUIDEBOOK

I LOST THIRTY POUNDS IN NINETY DAYS
THE HEALTHY WAY. I AM NOW 44 POUNDS LIGHTER.

NO CRASH DIETS, NO PILLS, NO EXCUSES!

DEDICATION

This book is God inspired and dedicated to my son Brian M. Stevenson who sacrificed many years while I finished school. Thanks to my brother Joseph J. Jimason who has helped me to realize my dreams, however many times I have started over. A special thanks to my family for all their support. I love them all deeply and will always be grateful for their kindness.

This book is also dedicated to all of you who have given up hope of ever losing weight. It can be done. You will learn to do what you thought was impossible to do…lose weight again.

CONTENTS

Introduction....What is Fat To Fit At Fifty +? vii

Part One: A Need For Change ix

1 My Story: Change Was Inevitable 1

2 No Excuses: Save Your Life 9

3 Free Yourself from Mental Garbage 13

4 Getting Motivated 19

Part Two: The Plan 25

5 The Plan: Support, Exercise, Food 27

6 Pitfalls to Avoid 39

7 Follow-Up and Resources 43

INTRODUCTION

My body had been invaded by some alien being and I needed to take back the occupied space. What I viewed in the mirror was foreign to me and unwanted. I no longer recognized the woman in the mirror staring back at me, an obese vegetarian trying to lose weight. With hope and a promise from God I got it done, I delivered a knockout punch to weight.

What is *Fat to Fit at Fifty+*? It is a **guidebook** that focuses on the emotional and mental barriers that can sabotage any attempt to lose weight, a no-excuses guidebook to help you lose weight the healthy way in a reasonable amount of time. It is a no-crash diet to losing weight without gaining it all back approach. There is no need to starve yourself or use any other crazy method that is simply not healthy for you. It is an overall wellness approach to weight loss.

What *Fat to Fit at Fifty+* is **not** is another book filled with diet plans and exercise programs—anyone can write a book and put in hundreds of diet and exercise plans that you will find on the Internet. It's also not a magic diet plan to follow as a way to fix your weight problems. *Fat to Fit at Fifty+* starts at the core of the problem. It starts with how we think and feel, our emotional and mental attachment to weight loss. This book is for all the repeat offenders who cycle through one diet program after another. Yes, you may get temporary results with some diet plans but then gain it all back. You then realize that your body is not going back to what it used to be, and age is no longer on your side. It's not so easy to drop ten pounds in one week like you once did when you were twenty-two years old. Those ten pounds take you more than a month to drop. You give up in frustration and reach for the desserts and junk food—and the cycle continues. Stop it!

Now the onslaught of health problems begins or worsens. Your doctor tells you that losing weight is necessary to control your illness. What your doctor is saying is that your health problems are largely food related, and you need to look at what you are putting in your body. Once again you think of how much you want to get rid of the weight and make a half-hearted commitment to begin yet another diet. You search the Internet for days and weeks looking for that one plan that will provide that quick and easy fix to your weight-loss problem. You find there are hundreds more diets added to the list of diets since the last time you searched. All the weight-loss fads out there are still promising that miracle. They show pictures of overweight people who supposedly lost one hundred pounds in sixty days and you wish that were you with the weight loss story. It's not them either unless they have been on some television program with a team of experts assisting and having them work hard all day long. Come on, deep within you know that they are selling you false hopes and dreams, but you are so desperate you decide to try the promised quick fix one more time. Don't do it! Those plans don't work for the long term.

Let me tell you that there is no easy method. Losing weight takes determination and a lot of hard work. The approach taken in the *Fat to Fit at Fifty+* is a sensible and healthy weight-loss approach. There are two rules you must follow: (1) you must eat, and (2) you must move your behind to drop pounds and keep them off. You don't want to get through this process only to find you traded weight loss for irreparable damage to your body because you ate too little or not at all. I will tell you some pitfalls to avoid and why this style of losing weight is not good for you to attempt.

So if you are truly fed up, ready to stop hiding and drowning in weight-loss misery, then let's get started. I will share my story with you as a warning about some of the main pitfalls to avoid. I will break down the steps to weight-loss success. Let me help you right now begin your weight-loss program.

Ready? Okay. Stand up and just walk in place for one minute. Do it! It may feel silly but it is the small steps and follow-through like this that will guarantee your success. I'm not joking. Get up right now and move your behind! If you did, then you are already on your way to weight-loss victory.

PART ONE

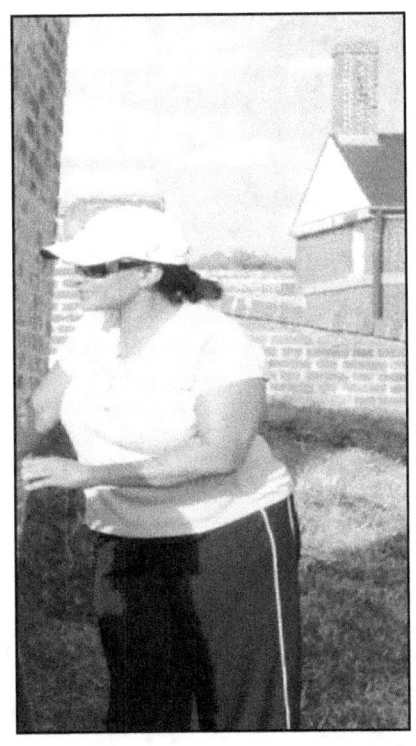

A NEED FOR CHANGE

CHAPTER 1

MY STORY

CHANGE WAS INEVITABLE

Mid-fifties, overweight, and worn from life, I suffered knee pain, back pain, and persistent aches. I experienced a rare stroke a year prior to my weight-loss journey and was unable to do any exercise. It was frustrating and derailed any motivation I had for change.

I had been through many life stressors over a seven year period and ultimately had an economic tsunami hit my life and wash everything I possessed out to sea. When the waves of life placed me back on shore with sand in my mouth, I had to get up and brush myself off to face the wreckage. I was left with nothing and had to make tough decisions about how to rebuild my life. My plan after losing my job through a company layoff and after nearly exhausting all savings including retirement savings, was to sell what I could and go to the East Coast. Jobs had dried up in California, the state was on the verge of bankruptcy and so was I.

By the summer of 2008, I relocated to the D.C. area, leaving my college-age son to move in with his father for the first time in his life. I left him with the promise that I would return as soon as the job market turned around in California. Well, we all know what happened to the economy during 2008 and it was not just in California; it crashed!

Please know that life is not always kind but you must not give up. If you stand up again, I promise that you will be stronger and more determined than ever to overcome your struggles. This is exactly what the weight-loss challenge is, a very tough struggle that you must overcome. Wipe the dust off, and start again.

Soon after moving east with family, I was fortunate enough to get job interviews and by the winter landed an interview where they were excited to hire. This was great! Before I could take advantage of any possible opportunity I suffered a brain hemorrhage, a rare form of a stroke. Doctors told me that it was not due to other health issues that are generally associated with a stroke, such as high blood pressure, diabetes, obesity, etc.

Doctors informed me that the type of stroke I experienced was rare in terms of where it originated, which was directly in the brain. I also learned that there was not very much the scientific world knew about this type of stroke. Belief among the medical community was that, in some cases, it could be faulty wiring of blood vessels at birth. They did not really know nor could they locate the actual area where the blood was leaking into my brain. They could only see that my brain was hemorrhaging.

This all started in December 2008 while I was preparing for the holiday festivities. My brother and his wife were having a gathering of family and friends for a pre-Christmas party, and I was creating music for this event. We had dinner, played games, and had a great time before deciding to call it a night.

While preparing for bed I was suddenly hit with tremendous pressure in my head, and the worst headache I had ever experienced in my life. Believe me, I knew headaches having made many visits to the emergency room for migraines that rendered me helpless. I shared with my brother what I was experiencing and that I was going to lie down to see if it would subside. As I walked towards my room, my legs went limp, and I became violently ill. I tried to speak but my speech was so slurred no one could understand me. Fortunately for me, my older brother recognized this symptom as being related to a stroke, and he immediately called for an ambulance.

In less than an hour, I awakened to find myself in the local hospital. I was told that I had bleeding in my brain, a stroke, and needed to be transported to a hospital better equipped to handle such a critical issue. In disbelief, I stated that there was no way that I could have had a stroke. I felt that they must be mistaken and inquired about the part of the brain that had been impacted, if any area had been at all. Before I could get that answer, I lost consciousness and woke up to someone standing over me who I later learned was my treating physician.

He recognized the seriousness of my situation and made some medical decisions that ultimately saved my life that night. He told me I was really sick. "I know you don't think so, but you are very sick," he stated. I did not have the energy to tell who I thought was a clerk or assistant at the time to get away from me with that madness. Later I mustered up the energy to ask what part of my brain was impacted. When I learned the area was in the base of my brain, which is the life center and controls breathing, I knew then that I was in danger and that possibly I would not survive. It was humbling.

When my family was informed that a hospital bed had become available in D.C. and that I would have to be transported by helicopter to get there, I then became fearful. I begged my brother to drive me because there had been a major medivac (medical transportation by air) in recent months, and I was afraid to chance riding with them. I begged and pleaded to no avail, "they've crashed 50% of the time" I stated. They drugged me and put me on the helicopter which transported me to a reputable hospital in the District of Columbia. My family called my son in California to come be with me due to the uncertainty of the outcome. I can't tell you how upset I was with them because I did not want him to drop classes in school to come be with me. I had never seen my son weep and it was all I could do not to breakdown with him. I made him crawl in my small hospital bed with me and held him like he was two years old. A sense of calm came over me and I assured him that I was not afraid of the outcome. I told him to allow them to do the surgery if necessary and gave him the name of my insurance agent in the event the outcome was not what we hoped.

They performed a microscopic procedure to locate the bleed and repair the vessel. To their surprise they could not find the ruptured vessel and it had actually stopped bleeding. I later inquired if my previous migraines were a factor or possibly stress related as I mentioned earlier that I had been through numerous life-altering events within the last seven years. Doctors told me with certainty that those issues were unrelated to my brain hemorrhage. I still doubt that assessment.

I had learned years earlier that migraines are partly food related. There are foods that contain tyramine such as chocolate, bananas, yogurt, cheese, red wine, mushrooms, etc., that can trigger migraines. Pretty much any food that requires aging can be a trigger. It really matters what you put in your body as it has a direct correlation with your health and how you feel.

Before being discharged from the hospital I was approached by researchers and asked to participate in a five-year study, and I agreed. The last follow-up at the three-year mark, I was told my brain showed no signs that anything had ever happened. This was good news.

It took one year for me to completely return to normal functioning, but I was blessed since I had walked away without any lasting disabilities. It was odd to me that only my senses were impacted. They were all heightened except for my sight. I could not see clearly even with glasses for a short period of time. My hearing, taste, touch, and smell were intensified. All sounds were louder, people's normal speaking voices sent me ducking under a pillow to decrease the volume. All sweet tasting foods were too sweet, salty foods were too salty, etc., but all eventually returned to normal.

I am grateful that I received some of the best care from beginning to end from all the medical staff and facilities that were involved in my treatment. I believe that is why I am alive today; God placed me in the best medical hands in the area. Research shows that a small percentage of the population experiences the type of stroke I had, and even a smaller percentage survive. It was also rare to survive without long-term problems or a disability. I was truly blessed to escape death. Even still, I knew I needed to change my lifestyle in order to avoid anything that closely resembled this narrow escape. I needed to lose weight and really focus on overall wellness, particularly since diabetes and high blood pressure were a part of my family's medical history. I felt that eventually these diseases would catch up with me if I didn't change my behaviors around food and exercise.

"Why was this was my portion in life?" I asked God. "Why so much pain over the years for what seemed to be a lifetime?" What escaped me was that if I had not been with family that night, I would have gone to bed to sleep off the headache and would have never awakened. My doctor said that there is a one-hour window for the best outcome for survival. Another point on the upside of my fragile life was that during this painful time, I paid down more debt in a short period of time not working than I would have been able to do while working full time. I also grew stronger emotionally and mentally, faced with decisions and life changes that I would have never had to address as a working person. So life dealt me lemons, and through God I made sweet savory lemonade.

I pray you never go through the years of struggles I have faced, but if you do, then try to find your blessing in all of it. You are stronger than you imagine, and you can overcome life storms. If you thought you were done, if you have stopped believing, I hope you draw strength and encouragement from my story to push through and start again. Use this type of strength to have your weight-loss breakthrough. Start to address your health issues by beginning your wellness program today. Have I said "now," or "today" enough? Good. You will see it more as you read. It is so critical to begin making a change immediately.

SUMMARY

- Don't wait for some life-altering illness to force you to change.
- Make you a priority, and take control of your health by starting right now on your path to wellness.
- Approach your wellness program with a sense of urgency.

Every day you wait the harder it gets and more importantly the harder it gets to drop the weight later. But I am here to give you the good news that if you start you will see positive results. And, if you start and stay consistent for a short period of time the benefits will last you a very long time. I preface this with the fact that once you have success at being healthy you will want to continue to be that way. You really lose the desire to eat like you did before. Your body hungers for healthy food, that's the great news. Your body actually helps you stay on track.

CHAPTER 2

NO EXCUSES

SAVE YOUR LIFE

That's right, no excuses! And don't surround yourself with people who make excuses because it will only validate your negative thinking and approach to weight loss. I know this because there were always people telling me that I looked okay. They were only comparing me to themselves or other heavier people. You cannot use others unhealthy physiques as a measure to determine if you should lose weight. At this point in your life you know you don't feel as good as you used to feel or look as good as you once did. You don't need others' affirmation to stay unhealthy. Listen to your own voice on your health and wellness and make the necessary change.

I am not telling you something that I did not experience myself. When I moved to the East Coast the weight I had started to gain seemed minor compared to the weight of others I would see in my community. In fact, I was considered small by comparison. Being heavy seemed to be the norm and I had room to grow to catch up with the norm. I continued to soak in my misery and destruction of my body with unhealthy nutrition and lack of exercise. Before I knew it I was no longer ten or twenty pounds overweight. I was now more than forty pounds overweight and dying a little each day.

I did not recognize the woman staring back at me in the mirror. When you have been a small person for most of your life and become heavy, it seems as though the battle is twice as hard. You are now dealing with a wounded ego, pride, and low self-esteem. You tell yourself that it does not matter and that looks are not that important, and yet you die each time you have to see someone you have not seen in a long time or anyone for that matter. What I learned through this experience is that it is not just about how you look. It is being the healthiest you can be right now in your life. Looking cute is the extra benefit.

I had so many excuses not to succeed. So when others would validate my excuses by agreeing that my battles were hard and that I had many reasons to be unsuccessful at my weight-loss dreams I felt somewhat comforted. However, I knew deep within that I was wrong and they were wrong for supporting my unhealthy behaviors.

You could have placed every excuse possible in a hat and pulled them out one by one, and I could identify with each and every one of them. It seemed I had them all and allowed those excuses to get in the way of my losing weight or starting a weight-loss plan. I needed a miracle!

What is your excuse? Tell me, what excuses are you using? Is it your age? Do you have knee and joint pain? Suffering from meno-pause symptoms? Too busy with the kids? Genetics? Health issues? Finances? What? Just name it, I have heard and experienced them all. They may be valid reasons to consider when approaching any new endeavor however they cannot be used as the reason to stay unhealthy. You cannot allow any reason to interfere with your weight-loss goals.

I began to exercise, testing my body and endurance with brief interval routines. Okay, initially I could only walk and not jog or run so I would push myself by increasing the incline on the treadmill for thirty seconds, then one minute, and so on until my body adapted.

Your body will adjust and you will find you are no longer winded with your efforts. Now when you reach your initial goals don't think "Good, I'll just stay here now that this is a   comfortable workout." No way. You now need to increase your time or your effort, speed up your walk, or try to run for thirty seconds, etc. Eventually you will be able to do this without much effort.

Get the picture? You are always exercising at the level you can handle all the while incorporating small sprints of intense exercise for brief periods of time to further push yourself. When you exercise this way your body begins to do more than you thought it could do, and the process gets easier. Don't tell me you can't do brief sprints because I am here to tell you that you can and will do them. This is exactly what I did with all the same complications that you have if not more.

SUMMARY

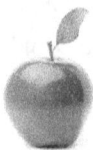

- Don't allow any of the reasons you felt were issues for starting weight loss to keep you from moving forward right now.
- Just start and watch your body aches lessen with exercise.
- Give it time.
- Don't surround yourself with people who are negative or who support your negative approach to getting healthy.
- Stop comparing yourself to other people and be the best you.
- Begin to come out of your hopeless state by taking the first step now. Right now, today, get up, and go for a ten-minute walk.

Remember this is your new beginning. Take small, baby steps. You can applaud yourself for your success. In the next week or two you will walk for twenty to thirty minutes and like it. You will continue to build from this point.

CHAPTER 3

FREE YOURSELF FROM MENTAL GARBAGE

T he biggest challenge is negative thinking and negative self-talk. We say awful things to ourselves that keep us stuck in a mindset of defeat. Stop it! You can talk yourself into an early grave or you can speak success and wellness over your situation. Really, don't you find that when you focus so much on a situation that it tends to happen, especially if it is negative? You have to think more positively about what you want for your life, within reason of course. You can't just think it you have to also act to make it happen. You can begin to lose weight by changing how you think about weight loss and then by changing your mind-set and then your behavior.

If you can move you can lose weight. All it takes is that initial effort and consistency to start your weight loss journey. This is called **discipline**. Discipline is something we all need to practice on a regular basis in order to master it. It takes a lot of discipline to be successful at weight loss particularly if you have tried over and over again without success. You must eat healthy and exercise. You can have weight loss with dieting only however it is a much longer process and does not address the need for you to build your body muscle and strength. You will need a strong frame to maintain overall health and to keep the weight off. A friend of mine who is also a nurse stated how important this is as it becomes increasingly important as you age in terms of maintaining independence and mobility. The best plan is clean eating, exercise, and managing stress.

Just like we have to move our bodies to build strong muscle and strength, we also have to exercise emotional discipline to build mental muscle. You have to dig deep to deliver a knockout to negative thoughts and negative input from people who say you won't and can't accomplish your weight-loss goals.

There will be mental barriers that can prevent you from starting your journey to wellness. I realized that it was not only discipline needed around my eating habits but it was also a need to address and tear down the mental roadblocks I placed in my own way. There were issues I allowed to prevent me from moving forward on losing weight. At times I even thought of how to adapt and accept living as an overweight person...really. I felt that it was too late in life for me to lose weight and that being thin again was something of the past. My weight in proportion to my height was considered obese. I told myself that I should just get over the idea of getting back to a size six or eight. I was so wrong in my thinking; this was self-induced mental battery. It was fear of failure that was choking my brain and drowning out any hope to healthy living.

These were the story lines that ran through my mind and kept me numb and incapable of change. It was a self-defeating mental attitude that put the brakes on making an effort to even try. Let me encourage you not to get stuck in your mental garbage. You will drown there if you accept the lies you feed yourself through doubt, fear, and negative thinking. You can feel as though no one understands where you are and how to help you. But know that you are not the only one who feels this way. I visited that dark place and almost lost my way there, so let me give you an expressway out of that mental torture.

The key is to refuse to accept these messages—even if you believe them act as though they are not your truth, because they are not your truth. Find something you really like to do, no matter how silly, and do it each time you think negatively. When you feel like this it takes a conscious effort to be happy so do what is needed to get to a positive place.

Okay, so I wasn't going to share my silly behaviors that got me through my process of weight loss, but a very special friend told me that I needed to "keep it real," and that others needed to hear what I did. So here it is. I would play music every chance I got—music from my Smartphone, from my iPod Shuffle, my laptop, my desk computer all day every day, anywhere and everywhere I could. It didn't stop there. I would always sing loud and most times off-key, but I didn't care because it felt good to me. It felt so good I would jump up and dance around the room, in the kitchen, the bathroom, walking to my car, in the store…really it became my escape from all negative thoughts and people. I danced and sang my way to being more than forty pounds lighter…I'm still dancing and singing. And, I am now working on building more muscle and getting a more toned body. Look out because you may see me one day in weight competitions, possibly.

I also took up dance and martial arts for fun. The first time I sparred in martial arts, I delivered a technical knockout three times in one minute on a male student who had studied martial arts for ten years and was many years younger than me. This is not to encourage you to go knock out people to lose weight, but you can deliver a knockout punch to the weight that's been kicking your behind for years by finding fun ways to exercise I temporarily put the gloves down to become a Pilates and Spin Instructor.

Let me help you change your thinking and thus your approach to weight loss. This is not for the faint of heart. It does not mean you can't faint but you must get back up and keep trying. Save your life, lose the weight in the next six months and see major progress in ninety days. Set healthy goals that are manageable for you but will also push you past your comfort zone. That is where the body gives in and starts to change. You will see a difference if you start. The key is to find what motivates you to change.

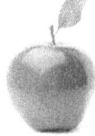

SUMMARY

- Push through negative thinking and self-talk.
- Find something that makes you smile (not food!), and use it every time you feel you are feeding yourself negativity.
- Actively work at discipline by building mental muscle. Turn your "I can't" into "I will," and then do it.
- Don't put off getting started because there will always be something that will keep you from moving forward.
- Plan and then start your wellness program.
- Stay consistent and begin with small steps so that you will have something to celebrate often.
- Don't allow yourself to be paralyzed with fear and hopelessness.

I have already shared my long list of issues that hindered my weight loss, and I could have continued to use them as excuses not to start this journey, but I did start and finished successfully. You can too.

CHAPTER 4

GETTING MOTIVATED

Please don't view this book or its approach as some new fad diet that hit the market. It is not! It is a fight for your life, your well-being while on this earth, a healthy guide to healthy living. I cannot emphasize enough how important it is to approach this from the standpoint of getting healthy. Looking cute comes as an end result of much hard work and yes, it is a great benefit but not the only reason to drop the weight.

There are enormous benefits to shedding those pounds; strengthening of bone, decreased symptoms of menopause, and the muscle aches and pains you thought you had to suffer each day will mostly disappear. The joint aches will also subside. If for no other reason lose the weight to get rid of the body pains you deal with every day or to eliminate the medications you take to reduce the pain.

When you are fed up with the joint pains, the isolation from the things you once loved to do, the slow dying inside and yet having to go on each day like all is well, you know it is time to make the commitment to change, today. Don't allow your life issues to sink you into a state of negativity or worse depression. You are living each day trapped inside a shell of a body that doesn't come close to sharing with the world the person you really are is simply a pity. Don't remain captive to your weight; don't continue to hide from the world. Unfortunately society is not kind about nor willing to overlook the overweight exterior frame we wear each day, but don't do this for others do it for you.

I used to look at myself and say that an alien being had landed in my body and overstayed its welcome. What I viewed in the mirror was foreign to me and unwanted. My body had been invaded, and I needed to take back the occupied space. I lost many battles but eventually won the war. It took planning, determination, emotional discipline and a willingness to act. It took God!

Right now I am urging you to make a decision to change. Take back your life and live again. Don't look at how long the journey is going to take or how long it's been. Just start. If you are anything like me, you need to see things in front of you in order to fully absorb them. So if you have to write down what you think stops you from becoming healthy emotionally, mentally, and physically, then write it down. However, don't spend a lot of time on this and forget to start the process. Just make some notes and then plan and act on your next step.

Given a Promise: A Power Greater Than Yourself

When presented with what seems to be impossible to overcome, I turn to God. He is my rock and my salvation, and I will forever trust in Him to carry me through difficult times; He is my motivation. This may not be true for some, but trust me you need a power greater than yourself to overcome some mountains in life. My mountain was being overweight and I needed God to show up to help me with the battle. So whatever power you need call on it and use it. It was this power, my God, my Christ that saved my life that year after a brain hemorrhage and who placed a team of excellent doctors around me. So I cried out to Him once more and He delivered.

I was trying every food plan that I could find on the Internet that promised to be healthy; juicing only, juicing and one meal, phase one of certain diet plans, meat and veggies only, etc. I saw weight loss of about fifteen pounds but within a few months put the pounds back on and more. I was so frustrated. One afternoon I decided to go to the park and walk. I plugged in my earphones to my iPod filled with praise songs and got started. As I walked and felt the breeze in my face I looked out at the green grass and deer feeding on the trees, and my spirit was lifted. I began to thank God for life itself and was brought to tears when I heard in my spirit God's promise to take away my desire for unhealthy eating and give me the physical strength to exercise if I would just start. Wow!

It was late summer/early fall and I was excited to make an effort to stand on this promise so I started walking a little more several times a week. At this point I was eating pretty healthily, had given up meats, and was leaning heavily toward being vegetarian. I did not attempt becoming a vegetarian for the sole purpose of helping with my weight-loss plan. I found that most meat textures did not sit well on my stomach. No, you don't have to be a vegetarian to follow this program or to lose weight. I later helped a client who at meat and she lost fourteen pounds in less than three weeks.

I was still snacking on cheese crackers, pretzels, you know… crunch food. What is it about food with crunch that gives you such satisfaction, such comfort? The weight was not moving. Now I was just an obese vegetarian trying to lose weight. This was more frustrating and embarrassing. You know people were looking at me saying, "Oh yeah? You are a vegetarian, huh?" I began to think that maybe I did not hear God correctly or even at all. Maybe I made it up because it was what I wanted to hear. I also know that you cannot doubt God or His promises as it is about faith and standing on His word. You must back up His promises with His word.

Read your Bible and if it isn't there then you can say it was made up. But if you can back up that promise with scripture then you can rest assured it was God speaking to you. So after reading the scriptures that supported God's desire for all to be healthy and healed, I felt certain that I had heard Him correctly that day in the park. I revisited His promise and re-evaluated what my part was in this journey. After all, He had just saved my life by what was considered to be very small odds. Certainly He could show me how to lose weight. I found healthy substitutes for crunch food (all different flavors of rice cakes) and soon lost all the desire for snack foods.

Again, your motivation may be something entirely different than mine but God works for me. I don't know what your most challenging life event has been but maybe you can draw from that experience. Maybe it has been several challenges that you have overcome. Good! This means you are strong and will have more to draw from to start your path to wellness.

Try to imagine what it took to overcome those challenges, imagine making those accomplishments, doing those difficult tasks you have done: giving birth, caring for an ill parent, overcoming financial hardships, or worse. Draw from any life-challenging event and ask if changing the way you eat is harder than that experience. This is exactly what I did. It works.

As a single parent it was challenging for me to get through graduate school. It was stressful having to get my son off to school at the exact same time I was due to be in my first class. So of course I would be late for my morning class by ten to fifteen minutes on those days I had to be there at 8:00 a.m. I remember my professor asking to see me after class. He looked at me and started by first telling me how he thought I was a "nice" person but that he had "some concern" about my commitment because I was often late for his class. All graduate students knew that on evaluations for grading your progress that "some concern" was serious and you were close to failing. I smiled and told him that it would not happen again and that I would correct the problem. He seemed so relieved and stated that he was impressed with my response. He was expecting excuses and a fight. I knew I was coming late so I offered no excuses.

So in this situation, it was not a question of my reasons why I could not be on time it was my responsibility and I simply took a no-excuses approach. I did not know at the time how I would work the problem out, but I knew I had to fix it. I was still rushing to pick up my son and finding care while I went to work at night. I came home and checked his homework or most times helped him complete the endless homework assignments. I am certain all you single parents out there can relate to trying to make your kid's sporting events, plays, teacher conferences, and sleepovers and how demanding coordinating all that can be. I had to call my retired brother on the East Coast and ask him to come live with me to help me out. He did not hesitate and was on the next plane it seemed.

Raising children particularly school-age children requires non-stop commitment, time, lots of effort, and more. However, that is another book in and of itself. The hours, days, and years of working hard as a parent to see our children get through school successfully would take many unrelated chapters to discuss. But as parents we do it. So you think we can change our behaviors around food and exercise? I think we can. Although, listing all that we do as parents may make you want to rush to the nearest ice-cream store...don't!

SUMMARY

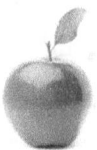

- Every time you think you can't eat healthily or exercise or commit to a wellness program just think of all you have already done, and use this as your motivation.
- Again, place the value on you and your health even if it means you have to be a little selfish in your approach. We can find so many reasons not to focus on ourselves due to taking care of something or someone else. You will not be there to help them if you don't change. As I said earlier if you need permission to become selfish with your time in order to get healthy then do so.
- Set aside time that is specifically for you to work on you.

Here is a word of caution: don't drop what you are doing in other areas and don't put the time into your wellness program. You will really feel depressed. So don't give yourself another reason to become frustrated. Take the time you need and really work on you.

PART 2

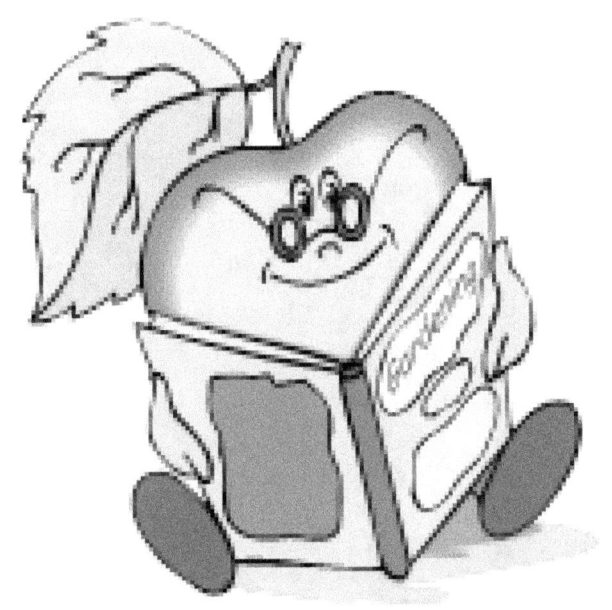

THE PLAN
Support, Exercise, Food

CHAPTER 5

THE PLAN

SUPPORT, EXERCISE, FOOD

I set goals and made sure to follow the plan. I took small steps each day to get on the right track. I tracked my progress so that I would have something to measure how far I had come. This is so important to do. Measure or track your progress, not just to have another task to do but to look at what you have accomplished when you feel you can't go any further. This will help you stay motivated.

I began to search for a gym that I could afford, where the cost was the absolute minimum or free. I spent time researching facilities within the community, such as nonprofit organizations, etc. until I found one. Within two days of the start of my search I was working out at a gym close to my home. Don't give up because it's too costly. There are some community agencies that may offer reduced fees. Whatever your financial stumbling block may be you can check your local community agencies, search the Internet, and negotiate terms with your local gym to get you started. Please don't let finances be the reason you don't start your program for weight loss. You cannot afford to do nothing. Now that's costly!

Choosing a Support System: Family and Friends Will Treat You Differently

This group is not necessarily your strongest support system when it comes to your weight-loss goals. You might do better finding an outside support group because those members may have the same goals you have to lose weight, and they will not judge you. I learned this the hard way. Some friends actually stopped communicating with me before and during my weight loss journey. It was uncomfortable for them that I had gone from a size six to an eight to a fourteen, so they avoided having to show their pity and disbelief by distancing themselves. I was okay with that as I did not want to be seen.

Through this process I learned who my friends were and trust me the list became very short very quickly.   For some reason being "fat" also meant to some that "stupid" came hand in hand with being overweight, or at least that is the way I thought they felt. In a sense I guess they were correct. How could anyone stay on a fast track to death? That is stupid.

Let me say this however, sometimes when we are in our own stuff and self-pity, small things can seem very big. When our opinion of our self is negative then we interpret what others are saying as negative as well.   Maybe it was a combination of both for me but it is a mind-set we cannot afford to wallow in too long. We simply cannot get stuck on what we think others are feeling about us, whether imagined or real. We need to keep the focus on our goals and the need to change our situation.

Now family God bless 'em, some of them will either support your being fat or they become so critical of you that all you want to do is find the biggest container of ice cream, dive in face first, and never come up, not even for air. You need something to make you feel better after interacting with them. Again, this may not be your support system! If they are you are blessed with a unique family.

Don't misunderstand my take on family support as they would be the first to show up and help me in any other area of my life and they have. However, my weight loss journey was not an area they could or even knew how to help. I was their baby sister and I looked just fine to them, after all I was "middle-aged" now and not expected to look like I did when I was younger.

At dinner one night with family and friends one family member looked at me and asked me when I was going to go running or something, implying that I needed to lose weight. You could hear a pin drop in the room. Everyone at the dinner table froze and tried to cover it up. At that point however, I had done some running and felt so good about my stamina that I challenged him to a race which was declined. I did not allow the comment to steal the joy of that night nor my plans to start my program. So I let it go unchallenged without making a scene. It also put the other guests at ease by keeping it light and not showing that the comment was offensive. You see if I didn't want to hear that kind of foolish talk then I had to keep working to lose the weight even if I felt the comment was completely out of line.

After I dropped the weight that family member still made no mention of my success. So you may not get the praise for your weight-loss accomplishment from those people who could only be critical of you for being overweight. But don't let that bother you. I think that they are so surprised you did it that they are simply speechless. I felt no one in my family thought I would ever be small again except my older brother who knew me well enough to know that when I made up my mind about anything I got it done. You just have to focus on you and let your results shut them all up.

So if you have a family or circle of people who have heard you say many times that you were going to drop the weight only to watch you gain pounds, then don't use them as support through this process—they no longer believe you and cannot support your efforts. Let this be the last time you declare your victory over weight. You can and will do this! Just follow the plan with consistency and you will succeed.

Find local walking groups to get involved with or online groups also striving to lose weight. This might be your best option if you have no other positive support system.

Choosing a Workout Plan

Always check with your doctor before starting any workout program. If you can hire a personal trainer from the start to guide you through a workout plan that keeps you safe then do so. However, if you cannot afford a trainer ask your gym to have someone train you on how to use the equipment properly. Don't assume you know. Many exercise routines that were once deemed safe to do on the machines have been revamped because they were not the safest way to use the equipment. So take the time and get that initial demonstration of proper equipment use

Get in lots of cardio workout at the start of your weight loss program. It is what burns fat and helps you drop pounds. The treadmill, elliptical machine, and stationary bikes are all great machines to help you start and build upon a workout that will fit you. You may start at a slow pace initially but soon find that you can go a lot faster and longer with less difficulty. Each time you acclimate to your exercise routine then it is time to change your pace. Don't cheat and stay on the same level because it feels good to you. Force yourself to make your workout challenging, or somewhat uncomfortable to complete, and always break a sweat. I would laugh at my sister who would say "I don't want to sweat." I would tell her she did not seriously want to lose weight. For some of us this means a real bad hair day but the payoff is so worth it.

When you start to see a drop in weight—a one-to-two-pound loss in your first week and the next couple of weeks to follow—start to incorporate some weight training. After approximately an eight-to-ten-pound weight drop, request to have a staff member at your gym show you how to use the weights properly. A staff member will never be as thorough with you as a personal trainer but take what the gym staff person offers for starters until you can do better on your own or when you can afford a trainer.

Here is what my workout plan looked like for the first 2 weeks of weight loss with a 5 pound weight drop;

My Two Week Workout Plan:

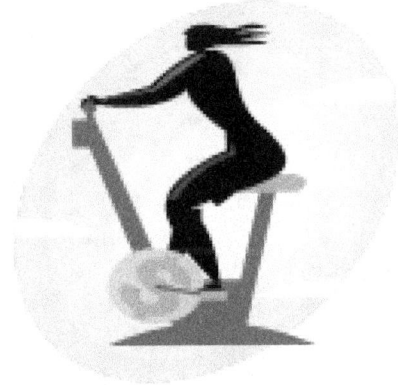

Days 1, 3, and 5 (Week 1)
30 minute walk on the treadmill varying speed:
3-5 minute warm up at 3.0
10 minute walk at 3.8
10 minute walk at 4.0
5 minute (cool down) walk at 2.0-2.5

30 Minutes on Elliptical Machine
Varying pace at what was comfortable

30 minutes on resistance equipment (get gym staff to show you how to use the machines)

Days 2, and 4
30 minute walk on the treadmill varying speed:
3-5 minute warm up at 3.0
10 minute walk at 3.8
10 minute walk at 4.0
5 minute (cool down) walk at 2.0-2.5

30 Minutes on Elliptical Machine
Varying pace at what was comfortable

60 minutes of Spin Cycling Class

Day 6
Rest

Day 7
60 minute Yoga Class (Stretch, Relaxation Style)

Days 8, 10,12 (Week 2)
30 minute walk on treadmill with gradual increase in incline, break down:
3-5 minute warm up at 3.0 speed, 3.0 incline
10 minute walk at 3.8 speed, 4.0 incline
10 minute walk at 4.0 speed, 5.0 incline
5 minute (cool down) walk at 2.0-2.5 speed, no incline
30 Minutes on Elliptical Machine
Varying pace at what was comfortable, increasing pace to running for 3-5 minutes twice within 30 minutes

30 minutes on resistance equipment (get gym staff to demonstrate how to use the machines)
Slightly increase the weight shown to you by a trained staff member of the gym

Days 9, and 11
30 minute walk on treadmill, break down:
3-5 minute warm up at 3.0 speed
10 minute walk at 3.8
10 minute walk at 4.0
5 minute (cool down) walk at 2.0-2.5
30 Minutes on Elliptical Machine
Varying pace at what was comfortable

60 minutes of Spin Cycling Class

Day 13
Rest

Day 14
60 minute Yoga Class (Stretch, Relaxation Style)

Try different equipment for cardio and weight training. Find what works for you and use variations to keep your body from becoming accustomed to the machines. Find a plan and stick with it for about two weeks, three weeks maximum then incorporate other equipment. Gradually increase the pace and duration at cardio.

SUMMARY

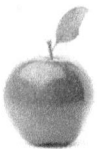

- Find a support system that is not judgmental of your desire to lose weight.
- Don't give up due to lack of finances as you can find resources through local community organizations.
- The key to your weight-loss success is consistency, consistency, and more consistency. And you must start now—no more putting it off until next year, next month, or the next day. If you need to break your workout into two sessions in a day, then do just that, but get in the time needed.

First you must exercise a minimum of four times per week for at least sixty to ninety minutes each time to see a change. Now don't get discouraged with this routine. It's only for the first ninety days of your plan and then you will want to start to monitor how much more weight, if any, you want to lose. Again, this is not easy but it is sure to work and it will also help you to keep weight off long-term. Secondly, you must simultaneously change your eating habits.

Food Choices

I'll preface this with check with your doctor before starting any change in your food intake, especially if you are under certain food restrictions or have food allergies. Use this as a start in your new eating habits however asks your doctor how you might substitute foods in the plan that may not work for you. Eat small meals 2-3 hours apart throughout the day (6 meals; breakfast then snack, lunch then snack, and dinner then a snack).

You must now start to eat clean. That means drinking lots of water and eliminating all processed and junk foods. Basically your diet will consist of meats, fruits, vegetables, whole grains, nuts, legumes, wheat pastas, brown rice, reduced dairy, etc. This way of eating is now your new best friend. Again, try this for ninety days and you are sure to see a big change in weight and how you feel. Surprisingly once you eat this way for a period of time you will begin to lose the desire for all the bad foods. Your body adjusts and no longer craves the junk.

The lists below consist of foods I ate during my initial weight loss program. Basically I stayed within 1400-1500 caloric intake per day based on what my body needed and for what my goals were at the time. You can find weight loss tools to determine what is best for you by doing an online search. I really liked Doctor Oz, Web MD, and Prevention for weight loss tools and meal plans.

My Two Week Food Plan (Vary Selections, Mix & Match), Choose One From Meal Choices

Breakfast Choices:

- Low fat yogurt, fruit, raisin bread or mini muffin
- Cereal (multigrain or plain Cheerios, any Fiber One, mix with Granola) with soy milk, fruit, pecan nuts, almonds
- Fresh Fruit Smoothie (Bananas, strawberries, blueberries, low fat yogurt, and cup of soy milk)
- Protein Shake

- Grits, 2 eggs, turkey bacon or veggie patty sausage
- Multigrain waffles with fresh fruit, light syrup
- Original oatmeal with fresh fruit
- Egg (fried in olive oil or boiled) and avocado sandwich (wheat sandwich thins)
  Coffee with soy milk (no sugar added)

Lunch Choices:

- Salad (Greek or Spinach)
- Lentil and Black Bean Soup, Mixed Vegetable
- Veggie Wrap
- Soy patty or links
- Protein Shake or Smoothie
- Vegetables, tofu, toasted lavas bread with pepper jack cheese
- Mushroom burger with humus, tomatoes, olives, carrots, or fresh salsa (one whole avocado, fresh salsa, squeeze fresh lemon and sea salt and mix) as spread or even as a salad dressing
- Fresh fruit salad, low fat yogurt
- Tofu, Quinoa, spinach

Dinner Choices:

- Portabella Mushroom burger with vegetables
- General Tsu Soy Chicken (vegetarian chicken), vegetables, brown rice or wheat pasta, and baked yam
- Stir fry vegetables, with tofu
- Spinach lasagna with salad
- Soy patty, potatoes, broccolini

All soy, tofu choices were matched with vegetables consisting of Bok Choy, spinach, broccoli, brussels sprouts, salads, broccolini, collard greens (try all vegetables)

Desserts:

Sugar free Jell-O, Greek yogurt mixed with dried cranberries and pecans, fresh fruit

Snacks:

Fresh fruit (apples, bananas, grapes, blueberries, strawberries, cherries, oranges, pears) dried cranberries, nuts (pecans, almonds), boiled eggs, veggies and salsa, low fat yogurt with cinnamon, flavored rice cakes for crunch food

Drinks:

- Four to six bottles of 16 oz waters per day
- Cranberry juice (limited)
- Coffee (unsweetened)
- Tea (green or black teas)

Breads:

Wheat sandwich thins, wheat wrap, pita pocket bread, lavas wrap, and mini wheat bagels

CHAPTER 6

PITFALLS TO AVOID

I promised to discuss some pitfalls to avoid, some that I personally experienced. I was so focused on my goals that I missed some key signs from my body. You must be mindful of your weight loss and make adjustments to your food intake as you lose. In other words, if your body weight calls for 2500 calories per day then be sure you are getting that amount of calories. As you burn up energy during your workout you will need this fuel to keep going without problems. If you do not give your body the nutrition it requires you will lose muscle, and at the end of your weight-loss journey you will look at a very saggy body. That's not what you want.

Also, if you are a vegetarian as I am now, then you must be aware of the pitfall of losing a significant amount of weight too rapidly. I did not realize that the body requires certain types of protein for overall health. I thought because I included some protein at each meal that I was okay with the amount of protein I consumed, but I was mistaken. The price I paid for this error was very slow muscle development and hair thinning. I lost about two-thirds of the thickness of my hair. It came out at the root and I was devastated! My hair did begin to grow in again but it was a challenge to get it back to normal.

I later learned that I needed to include supplemental protein such as shakes and specific foods high in protein to build muscle and keep strong hair and nails. There seems to be a debate in the vegetarian community as to whether you can build up muscle mass the same as meat eaters do. Some research articles found on the Internet state that it does take longer as a vegetarian to build muscle due to lack of animal protein. As long as you are getting an adequate amount of protein and incorporating weight training into your workout, there should be no problem with building muscle.

My trainer and I both realized that it was taking too long to see muscle form and that something else must be wrong. He told me I needed to eat meat or add more protein. I researched the issue and found that he was correct. I begin to drink protein shakes within one hour of completing my weight training. Studies show that protein is supposed to help to increase muscle and increase weight loss. In addition I needed to add more calories to my diet. After losing the weight and attempting to build muscle I needed to eat to compensate for the amount of energy burned at each workout session. So investigate these areas thoroughly, watch how your weight changes and make adjustments accordingly.

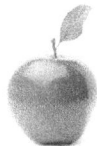

SUMMARY

- Reassess what your body needs as you make progress. As you meet each new goal, make certain you make the necessary adjustments.
- Be mindful of your caloric intake and make sure that it is adequate for your body weight and your physical output.
- Don't overlook the importance of additional protein in your diet as this has a direct impact on building muscle.
- Remember, due to inadequate protein and low food intake I had hair loss, so don't make the same mistake.
- Increase or decrease your cardio and weight training as needed. This step is so important. You don't want all your efforts to be in vain.

Don't sacrifice your total health for quick gains. As we get older muscle is much more difficult to build. When we don't eat and exercise properly we run the risk of losing muscle.

CHAPTER 7

FOLLOW-UP AND RESOURCES

It's challenging yet simple, but you can do this and be able to celebrate your success. If you have been following the plan discussed in this book as you read it then you will have something to celebrate right now. It may not be all the weight you want to lose but you are sure to be twenty to thirty pounds lighter. That's a great beginning but don't stop there. By now you must realize this is a lifestyle change. As I stated earlier this is not a fad-diet plan or a quick fix. This is a change-of-life guidebook to wellness.

Your focus should either be on continuing to lose weight or maintaining and firming up your new body. Keep going and remember consistency, consistency, consistency. You can and will be successful.

Resource Websites for Weight Loss:

www.doctoroz.com
www.webmd.com
www.prevention.com
www.sandraslifesecrets.com

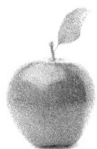

SUMMARY

- Celebrate your success
- Have fun while you exercise
- Don't quit, it's not an option

Celebrate what you have done. Continue if you need to lose more weight but make certain to assess the needs of your body as you make progress. Don't forget to incorporate toning and weight training. It's not enough just to be thin you want to also be strong.

Good luck on your weight-loss journey, and don't forget to have fun!